A WORTHWHILE DUTY

A book on keeping our body and mind
healthy because that is the way we show we
are grateful to Him for His Gift

DR RADIAH SALIM

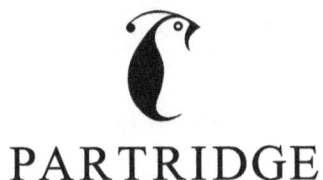

PARTRIDGE

Because of the dynamic nature of the Internet, any web addresses or links contained in this book may have changed since publication and may no longer be valid. The views expressed in this work are solely those of the author and do not necessarily reflect the views of the publisher, and the publisher hereby disclaims any responsibility for them.

Print information available on the last page.

To order additional copies of this book, contact
Toll Free +65 3165 7531 (Singapore)
Toll Free +60 3 3099 4412 (Malaysia)
orders.singapore@partridgepublishing.com

www.partridgepublishing.com/singapore

CONTENTS

"In loving memory of
Umi and Abah"

FOREWORD

Good health, both physically and mentally, is important for us to lead meaningful, fulfilling and happy lives. The value of good health becomes even more important as Singaporeans are living longer. We want to add not just years to our lives, but also life to our years.

uA Worthwhile Duty" is a useful and simple guide that empowers readers to take charge of their health. The book provides tips and insights that individuals can adopt to care for ourselves and our loved ones. Dr Radiah Salim also makes a crucial link between physical and mental health, and emphasises the importance of taking a more holistic approach towards health and wellness.

Looking after one's wellbeing impacts not just individuals, but also families and communities. I am therefore encouraged by the efforts of Club HEAL to promote good health and well-being in the community.

I hope that many will benefit from the insights and tips shored in this book.

Let's do our port to help raise awareness about the importance of mental health and reach out to support those with mental health issues so that they too can lead meaningful and fulfilling lives.

Halimah Yacob
Patron In Chief,Club HEAL
President of the Republic of Singapore
17 September 2019

PREFACE

"You have a duty to your body"
$\qquad$ *—{Hadith, Bukhari]*

Health takes many *forms*- physical, mental, emotional, social, financial and spiritual.

Usually though, when we speak of health, we refer to our physical well being. Many now realize physical health is interlinked with the other aspects. For example, when *a* person is mentally and emotionally healthy, he or she is more likely to be physically healthy. This is because a healthy mind will be able to reason well and positive emotions will help motivate *a* person to take the right steps towards *a* healthy lifestyle that is a prerequisite to physical health.

Social health is important because "no man is an island". We need other humans as company and as support to one another, beginning with the family unit.

Financial health is important too ... as the popular saying goes – "money is not everything but almost everything needs money".

The ultimate though is our spiritual wellbeing. How we view our relationship with the Creator of the Universe and our role in this temporary life will determine our intentions and, hence, our actions.

Prophet Muhammad (sow) said:

> *"You have a duty to your Lord, you have a duty to your body and you have a duty fa your family so give each one its rights."*
> –{*Hadith, Bukhari]*

I spent many years working at polyclinics in Singapore, where the flow of patients was practically unceasing. At the end of each working day,

I would be exhausted but satisfied that I had done what I could for my patients.

Occasionally, I would meet a middle-aged or elderly patient who hardly ever fell sick and had no chronic illness. Even as I admired them, it made me wish I had a smaller patient load. I would then have more time to share with ather patients facts about the human body so that they too could understand that it was possible to prevent chronic illnesses well into one's old age. Hopefully with the knowledge gained, patients will exercise more of the patience and discipline necessary to remain healthy.

The work of a family physician is not merely to treat minor health conditions or common chronic illnesses and to refer the rest to the emergency department or the specialist clinic. We are placed in an excellent position to empower our patients through our knowledge and experience. In fact, a doctor has a duty to educate his or her patients.

It is with this specific intention to share that I have embarked upon this project entitled "A Worthwhile Duty".

My fervent hope is that readers enjoy this book and find it useful.

> *"The best doctor gives the least medicine"*
> *—Benjamin Franklin*

CHAPTER 1

Actions are but by Intentions

*"Deeds are {measured] by intentions, and
an individual is [rewarded] according to what
he intends ..."*
　　　　　　　　—[Hadith, Bukhari]

We all know the rules *of* leading the perfectly healthy
life: eat moderately; exercise regularly; manage stress. But
many of us do not follow them. We wont to. We resolve
every New Year *to* do so. But one week later we fall bock
to our bod habits. Doctors *see* ever-increasing numbers
of patients in their clinics, most of them suffering from
chronic illnesses brought upon by lifestyle choices. That is
why, even before we change our lifestyle, we need to reflect
on our motivations. The proper motivation is likely to see
us through when we resolve to make changes in our life.

As a Muslim, our Prophet (saw) has taught us that deeds
ore evaluated by our intentions. If we perform deeds

for the sake of seeking Allah's pleasure, then we will be motivated to continue performing them because we believe we will be reworded for it. That is why, as Muslims, we pray five times a day and we fast during Romodhon regardless whether it is easy or not. There is no question of giving up on our resolution in the middle of the year or the middle of Romodhon.

On the other hand, if what we do is for worldly gain, we will continue to oct only as long as our efforts yield worldly gain. When our objective is to amass huge sums of money or the approval of some people, we may never hove enough of either. In the process, we ore likely to ignore our health. We may evan and up cheating or oppressing others, or we may feel the outcomes ore not worth the effort, and we give up. Regardless of the outcome, we ore almost certainly going to be reworded with little lasting satisfaction.

When we do things for the sake of Allah and His Messenger, every action we do is transformed to on oct of worship. And when we worship Him, we know that the reword of God is **assured** and **unlimited,** so we ore more likely to be motivated to persevere and exercise core in what we do.

Hence the trick to o lasting change in our lifestyle is to recognise that our body is on *amanah* (a trust) given to us by God. We have a duty to keep our body and mind healthy because that is the way we show we are grateful to Him for His **gift.**

CHAPTER 2

Anxiety

The start of many illnesses both chronic and acute

"If anyone continually asks pardon, Allah will appoint for him a way out of every distress, and a relief from every anxiety, and will provide for him from sources he cannot imagine."
— {Hadith, Abu Dawood}

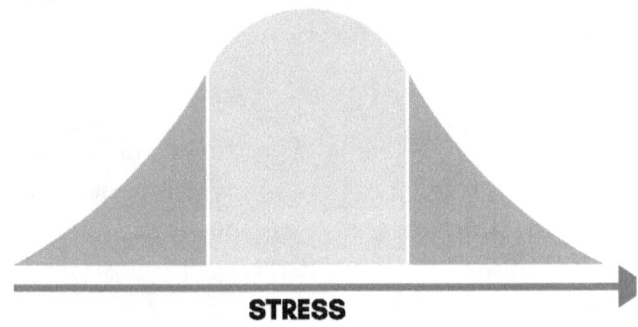

STRESS

I still remember when I was studying in junior college, one of my teachers explained the bell-shaped curve of performance versus stress as follows:

PERFORMANCE

In short, stress is important for us to achieve peak performance, but when one is overly stressed, performance declines.

Some anxiety is actually useful because it stimulates the brain to release the hormones that keep us alert and driven. It allows the student to push herself just a little more because she wants to excel in her exam. It allows the car driver to watch out for every traffic signal and for jay walkers, keeping him and others safe on the road. It provides both participants and spectators the thrilling feeling in a competition.

Too much of the stress hormones- adrenaline and cortisol - however, can lead to serious problems.

Adrenaline makes us more alert, but too much of it con give us sleepless nights. It con also cause o rise in blood pressure, give us sweaty palms and cause fatigue.

Cortisol, on the other hand, causes a rise in blood glucose levels, which can be useful when we need more energy. Too much of it, however, lowers our immunity against infection. Hence, it con trigger o host of acute conditions such as upper respiratory tract infections (including the common cold and influenza), tension headaches, gastritis, as well as chronic conditions such as hypertension, depression, diabetes and eczema. This is why many students fall sick during the exam season or experience o flare-up of their eczema.

Furthermore, developing one chronic condition may lead to developing another. For example, people with diabetes who are overstressed may develop depression. This can make them ignore their health, which usually corresponds to o worsening of their diabetes, leading to complications such os kidney failure or blindness.

On the other hand, I have seen some of my patients with hypertension improve when they leave their stressful jobs. Some eventually go off their medications.

Therefore, when you go into **sympathetic overdrive,** you literally become 'sick with worry'. When the stress is lessened, people improve.

Wouldn't it be nice if we can manage our stress levels so that we can prevent this domino effect, i.e., ovoid the onset of a chronic illness?

CHAPTER 3

Genetic Predisposition

"It is He who forms you in the wombs however He wills. There is no deity except Him, the Exalted in Might, the Wise."
−{Ouran 3:6]

Health conditions tend to run in families because of the genes we inherit from our parents.

In my family, we have members with diabetes, cancer, hypertension and mental illness. When overstressed, there is a risk we will develop one or more of these illnesses.

One of my in-laws has asthma, allergic rhinitis and eczema in her family line. The affected members have "atopy" - they are hypersensitive to allergens such as house dust mites, pollen and sweat. Her three daughters all have at least one of these conditions. My niece with eczema has flare-ups when stressed during exam periods, as the adrenaline rushes causes her to perspire more, and sweat irritates her skin and worsens the eczema.

Everyone has the potential to develop anxiety, depression and eventually psychosis if overly stressed, but genes can increase one's risk. Teenage and young adult years, especially, can be very stressful. This is why many people with o family history of mental illness first manifest symptoms during adolescence or early adulthood.

In short, the kind of illness we ore more likely to develop depends on our genetic predisposition. While we cannot choose our genes, we can manage our lifestyle so as to reduce the likelihood of those illnesses manifesting themselves. At the very least, our actions con reduce the extent to which the illnesses affect our lives.

And the first step in the right direction is to manage stress.

CHAPTER 4

Why We Get Stressed

our worldly goods and your children are but
a trial and a temptation, whereas with God
there is a tremendous reward."
—*[Our an 64:15]*

There are three main reasons why people get stressed:

- Chasing the material
- Needing to live up to the expectations of others
- Fear of death

Chasing the material

6/ am a material girl, in a material world"
—*Madonna*

"Material" includes money, big houses, fancy cars, grand titles, good looking life partners, cute and high-achieving children, and wonderful holidays to Europe.

We think we need these to achieve happiness because we have been conditioned to aspire to these goals when we were young. Surely all of us have heard some version of the following advice as the reason to study hard:"If you get good grades, you can go to university. You need a degree to get a well-paying job. After that you can get a handsome [or pretty] husband [or wife], buy a big house and drive a big car. Then you and your children can always be happy."

Pursuing the material is not wrong in itself, but life is not always as smooth-sailing as we want it to be. If we tell ourselves that we need to achieve all the above to be happy, not achieving just one of these can make us feel like failures. Worse, the rare individual who achieves all these will likely be disappointed- as if something is still missing.

It is human nature to crave and covet.

But there is a remedy: When we instil in ourselves a sense of gratitude and appreciation, we can overcome this human failing.

Living up to the expectations of others

Frequently, we chose the material because we wish to impress others. We worry a lot about what others- our parents, relatives, friends, even strangers- think of us.

We crave approval, so we do things that we know are not good for our health just to please others.

Our choice of study, work and even spouse is often influenced by how these will affect our standing in society, not because they truly give us happiness.

This leads to long-term stress that will inevitably lead to depression and illness.

The remedy: We need to know what we really need in life to be happy.

Fear of death

Last but not least, the thought of growing old and frail and dying is a very scary prospect for many, especially for people who do well materially, because all the money in the world cannot buy us eternal life.

Fear of death is fear of the unknown.

What would happen to me if I die ... will/ just rot and get eaten by the creepy crawlies?

Will anyone ever remember me?

Will my family be happier if I die, as they can then inherit my wealth? What if there is an accounting after death ... will I be tortured in the grave and in hell?

No, I am not ready to die.

Fear of death stops folks from doing brave things such as fighting for their country, or reaching out to people in war and disaster zones because of hazardous conditions, leaving victims of war and disasters to fend for themselves.

The person who is preoccupied with the fear of death can never be well.

In contrast, for a believer, death is a beautiful beginning to the next world!

> .... *Indeed, to Allah we belong, and to Him is our return ...*
>
> −{*Ouran 2:156*}

CHAPTER 5

Success Redefined

"Remain, then, conscious of God as best you can, and listen (to Him), and obey (Him). And spend in charity for your own good: whoever is saved from their own greed, indeed, they are the ones who reach a happy state!n
−{Our' an 64:16}

To ovoid the undue stress that accompanies the chose of the material, we would do well to reflect on what constitutes real success.

A good friend of mine, Ustozoh Loilo Abu Hasan, volunteers with Club HEAL, on organisation that assists people with mental health issues in their recovery journeys. She makes the participants of Club HEAL's rehabilitative programme repeat after her as follows:

"I om happy! I om healthy! I om wealthy!"

Notice that happiness comes **before** health and wealth, and not vice

versa.

Happiness is the true measure of success, because only with that will health and wealth translate into meaningful successes. Seeking material success to achieve happiness is therefore *a* big mistake, as it puts the cart before the horse.

What then con make *a* person happy?

Recent studies hove backed up the Our'onic message that helping others is *a* guaranteed way to achieve happiness:

> *If anything, it appears that there is a relationship between non materialism and well-being. While possessing wealth and material goods doesn't lead to happiness, giVmg them away actually does. Generosity is strongly associated with well-being. For example, studies of people who practice volunteering have shown that they have better psychological and mental health and increased longevity.*
>
> *The benefits of volunteering have been found to be greater than taking up exercise, or attending religious services – in fact, even greater than giving up smoking. Another*

> *study found that, when people were given a*
> *sum of money, they gained more well-being if*
> *they spent it on other people, or gave it away,*
> *rather than spending it on themselves ...*"
> —*Steve Taylor Ph.D,*
> *Psychology Today (9 January 2015)*

For me personally, my greatest success was the honour and privilege I enjoyed in caring for my late mother while she was alive, particularly during her last days. I can never repay the debt I owe Umi for being my mother. Nevertheless, it was wonderful to be "The Chosen One" from among seven siblings!

CHAPTER 6

Healthy Lifestyle

"The deeds *most loved by God (are those) done regularly,* even *if they are few."*
— [Hadith, Bulchari}

Avoiding prolonged and repeated stress is one aspect of preventing illness. The other aspect is choosing to live healthily. A healthy lifestyle encompasses a few deliberate choices with respect to diet, work/study and exercise, as well as sleep, rest and leisure. A healthy lifestyle is imperative for the prevention of any illness.

And then we need to have the discipline to regularly act on these few choices.

Discipline refers to training oneself to do something in a controlled and habitual way, for example, sleeping early at night and getting up early every morning, or exercising for half an hour daily.

Most of us already know what the healthier choices are, but we fail to practice a healthy lifestyle due to ingrained bad habits and the inability to discipline ourselves to make the necessary changes. We succumb to inner desires and outward pressure (from close friends as well as irresponsible media, such as advertisements) that encourage unhealthy choices.

> *"... they only follow their own lusts. And who is more astray than one who follows his own lusts, without guidance from God ..."*
> −{*Ouran 28:50*}

BUT, change is POSSIBLE!

You can develop the discipline to reclaim your health when Allah is there to help you, so try the following:

- *Remember your goal:* you will not only feel better but also please Him by the effort you put into improving your lives.
- Make a list of what healthy habits you need to implement and what negative ones you need to remove.
- Choose one or two habits to work on, and strive to keep at it for a month.
- Begin with Bismilloh whenever you oct on the habit – as with any other oct of worship.
- Renew your *niyyat* {intention) to continue with these habits every morning – remember you ore doing this for Allah.

- After a month of acting on the above, start a new cycle with on additional new habit from your list.

  ":.. Indeed, Allah will not change the condition of a people until they change what is in themselves ..."

  $-\{Ouran\ 13:11\}$

CHAPTER 7

Nutrition and Fasting

"There is no vessel which the son of Adam can fill with evil more than his stomach, for it is sufficient for him to take a few mouthfuls in order to straighten his back; but if he must, then fill one-third with food, one third with drink, and one-third with breath."
—[Hadith, Ibn Majah]

'When one of you is fasting, he should break his fast with dates; but if he cannot get any, then (he should break his fast) with water, for water is purifying."
—{Hadith, Abu Dawood}

Discipline in making- and staying with- good dietary choices will go a long way in maintaining good health and beating stress.

There are a few general principles to observe:

- Slight hunger is better than over-eating.
- Eat wisely.
- Drink water.

Slight hunger is beHer than over-eating

> *"Deeds are shown (to Allah} on Mondays and Thursdays, and /like my deeds to be shown when I am fasting."*
> —*[Hadith, Tirmidzi]*

Fasting does not just give us spiritual benefits –the physical benefits are scientifically documented as well. When fasting, our blood glucose dips. The body then turns to glucose stored in the liver and muscles to carry out our daily activities. This begins around eight hours after the last meal is consumed. When the stored glucose is used up, the body will burn stored fat for energy, which will result in weight loss. The use of fat for energy also helps preserve muscle mass and reduce cholesterol levels. Additionally, toxins stored in the body's fat are dissolved and removed from the body when fat is burned. Also, after a few days of fasting, higher levels of endorphins - "feel-good" hormones - are produced in the blood. Hence, fasting not only detoxifies the body, it literally makes us feel better.

Caution: Intermittent fasting is not suitable for everyone. People who have eating disorders, who are underweight, individuals under the age of 18, pregnant women, people with type 1 diabetes and individuals recovering from surgery, should not fast without first consulting o doctor.

Eat wisely

The nutritional needs of someone depends on age, gender and nutrient needs. For example, a pregnant woman will need more folate, calcium and iron in her diet. Someone training for the marathon will need more carbohydrates. Nevertheless, some basic principles hold true for everyone.

Tjmjng

Always drink water and eat fruits before your main meal because they reduce hunger. Always have a good breakfast because it provides the energy you need after you hove been fasting through the night. Also, have an early dinner, because eating a meal just before sleeping increases the risk of developing gastro-oesophageal reflux disease (GERD).

8glgneed megls

- *More fruits and vegetables:* Leafy and non-starchy fruits and vegetables are better than sweet or starchy ones in preventing blood sugar spikes. They all contain fibre, which keeps the digestive system healthy, stabilises glucose and cholesterol, and prevents heart diseases and same types of cancer. Fruits and vegetables also come in many colours and provide vitamins, minerals that we need (aka phytonutrients) as well as antioxidants that help prevent cancer.

- *Less added salt and sugar:* While these add flavour to our food, too much of it can adversely affect your blood pressure and your weight.

- *Avoid trans (partially hydrogenated oil} and saturated fats:* Food made with trans-fat are less likely to spoil, so it is found commonly in commercially-prepared food and snacks, including pizzas and potato chips. Trans-fat is the worst type of fat it because it raises our "bad" cholesterol (LDL) and lowers our "good" cholesterol (HDL). A diet laden with trans-fat increases our risk of heart disease.

- *Choose monounsaturated fats:* When cooking, use oils like canola oil or olive oil. Nuts, fish and other foods containing unsaturated omega-3 fatty acids are good choices as foods with healthy fats.

- *Eat proteins in moderation:* While necessary for muscle building and growth, these should generally be no more than a quarter of our meal portion.

Drinkwater

Water is the best way to quench our thirst. Avoid fruit juices and soft drinks as they are laden with unnecessary calories and is the easiest way to diabetes.

This brings us to the topic of our next chapter- Water!

CHAPTER 8

Water

'We sent down water from the sky - blessed water with which We caused gardens to grow, groins for harvest, and toll palm-trees with their spathes piled one above the other, sustenance for Our servants. With that We gave (new) life to a dead land. Similar to that will be the emergence (from the tombs}."
−{Oulan 50:9-11}

Water- the source of life

Clean water is truly one of God's greatest gifts. Up to 65% of the human adult body is water.

Body composition varies according to gender and fitness level because fatty tissue contains less water than **lean** tissue.

Lock of water leads to dehydration, which increases the likelihood of developing kidney stones, gout (o painful joint condition due to high uric acid), headache and myalgia (muscle ache).

Without food it is possible to survive up to eight weeks, but without water, we will die within a week or less, depending on factors such as heat and activity level.

Many foods contain water, especially vegetables like lettuce, cucumbers and tomatoes. Including these generously in your meals is an easy way to ensure that you satisfy your hunger and remain hydrated, while keeping your calorie intake low.

Water- a wonderful medium for pain relief

The other use of water is in pain-relief. As we grow older, many of us develop osteoarthritis, the development of painful joints due to wear and tear. Swimming helps, but even if you cannot swim, simply wading in the water will help to relieve your painful joints and muscles around them.

Water is also essential for the maintenance of hygiene -the topic of our next chapter.

CHAPTER 9

Hygiene

"Oh you who believe, when you get up to observe the Sa/at (prayer}, wash your faces and your arms to the elbows, and wipe your heads, and your feet to the anIdes."

—[Quian 5:6]

Our skin provides a protection for our internal organs. It protects the body from bacteria, viruses and other unwonted substances. However, any breach of the skin from injury con result in serious infections and damage to our interior. Hence, it is important to maintain good skin health.

Unhygienic conditions con result in itch and when we scratch, we may break our skin barrier.

Lack of hygiene can also result in contaminated water and food supplies, which may result in serious infections such as gastroenteritis (inflammation of linings of stomach and intestines resulting in abdominal pain, vomiting and diarrhoea).

Singaporeans generally enjoy good health because we have easy access to clean water and sanitation, as well as an army of cleaners at every park, housing estate and eating outlet. These are truly blessings of God, Most Generous.

Nevertheless, germs are everywhere. The simple practice of handwashing before and after meals helps reduce gastroenteritis.

Also, weird as it may look to some, it is actually a good idea to use face masks in crowded places like the MRT during morning and evening peak hours, at least during times when your immunity is compromised; it can significantly reduce your chance of developing common upper respiratory tract infections.

> *"Water, air and cleanliness are the chief articles in my pharmacopoeia."*
> —*Napoleon Bonaparte*

CHAPTER 10

Apparel

"'0 Children of Adam! Wear your beautiful apparel at avery time and place of prayer: eat and drink: But waste not by excess, for Allah loveth not the wasters."

−{Oulan 7:31}

The human skin is not a sufficient barrier to the elements of wind, fire, earth and water. Other animals in the animal kingdom enjoy thick hair or fur, we do not. Appropriate clothing is therefore a necessity, not just for the sake of modesty, but also for added protection.

Exposed skin is also more vulnerable to developing dermatitis from chemicals, contracting diseases such as dengue due to mosquito or other insect bites, or suffering serious abrasions from falls or other types of contact injuries.

The type of material used for clothing can also impact us. Most comfortable and least likely to irritate our skin would be light cotton, especially in the hot tropical climate.

In cold weather, on the other hand, the lack of adequate warm clothing can result in hypothermia – a potentially serious condition. Less serious but also importantly, a person is more likely to get an upper respiratory tract infection such as the common cold or the flu, which has the potential to progress to pneumonia, simply due to inadequate clothing in cold weather.

Adequate footwear too is important. In parts of the world where children run around barefooted, the chances of contracting parasites such os the hookworm are greater.

The type of footwear also needs to be factored in. Wise is the person who sacrifices glamour for practicality. Many foot conditions, such as deformities and plantar fosciitis con be avoided, by wearing comfortable footwear with adequate space for the toes and support for the soles.

Yet, since God himself tells us to wear beautiful clothes in the Holy Our'on, this is o hint that nice clothes con hove o significant impact on our life. In short, the type of clothes we choose to wear is port of our personality and body image, and potentially o boost to our self-esteem -something that impacts our mental and emotional well-being.

Hence, let us be guided by all the above in making doily choices regarding our attire: let it help us look good and feel better!

CHAPTER 11

Exercise

*uA strong believer is better and more beloved
in the sight of Allah than a weak believer,
but there is good in both."*
—[Hadith, Muslim]

The benefits of exercise are immense. It improves our overall health in many ways. Physically, this includes controlling our weight and blood pressure, strengthening our bones and muscles, improving our insulin resistance (and hence improving our blood sugar levels) and immunity to infections, and helping us sleep better. Psychologically, it improves our endurance and resilience in the face of mental stress. If done in a group, it also helps strengthen bonds.

Exercise leads to the production of natural painkillers called endorphins. These produce the same pain-relieving effects as synthetic drugs, e.g., morphine and codeine.

Beneficial exercise is regular exercise. According to ActiveSG, an adult should exercise for at least 150 minutes every week of moderate physical activity (e.g., brisk walking), in 10 minutes (or longer) sessions. Exercising in the company of family and friends will make sticking to the regime easier.

Exercise can be categorised as follows:

- *Aerobic (endurance):* increases breathing and heart rate (e.g., brisk walking, jogging and dancing).
- *Strength:* strengthens muscles (e.g., lifting weights, push-ups and using resistance bands}.
- *Balance:* helps prevent falls (e.g., standing on one foot, heel-to-toe walk and ToiChi).
- *Flexibility:* stretches muscles and helps body stay supple {e.g., shoulder, upper arm and calf stretches and yoga).

Exercise con be worked into our doily routine with o little planning and creativity. Housework. and taking public transport such as the train or bus con easily translate into o form of exercise.

My home is o 10-minute brisk-walk away from the nearest train station, and within o month of giving up driving and using the train and bus, I reduced my weight by 2kg and improved my blood pressure readings. I also sleep better! In addition to reaping financial and health benefits, I om doing my port in reducing carbon emissions in Singapore, olhomdulilloh!

In Singapore, by God's grace, it is easy to start exercising even if you hove been o couch potato all your life. In addition to cheap and well equipped public gyms, there ore also many free exercise and gym clinics that you con sign up for to help you develop o new exercise regime- just check the government's ActiveSg initiatives.

As has been stressed earlier, first make the choice to exercise, then tailor that exercise according to your needs and constraints - but be consistent. The ActiveSg motto is opt and worth internolising:HBetter beats perfect". Start now and get better every day instead of planning to achieve o perfect exercise regime.

Indeed, exercise should be the first thing we do every morning as we stretch ourselves upon waking up after o refreshing night's sleep -the subject of our next chapter.

CHAPTER 12

Sleep

"And have made your sleep as a thing for rest."
−{*Qur an 78:9*}

Sleep is essential to protect the mental and physical health of an individual, in addition to improving the quality of life. During sleep, several important processes occur that support the healthy function of the brain and overall physical health.

For example, sleep helps to maintain the balance of hormones such as leptin (regulates feelings of hunger and fullness), which is why inadequate sleep increases one's risk of obesity. Other hormones such as insulin, responsible for the regulation of sugar in the blood, also change and can result in an increase in blood sugar level. Hence chronic sleep deficiency is also linked too higher risk of cardiovascular disease, stroke, diabetes and kidney disease.

Further, growth and development are intricately linked to sleep. Deep sleep helps boost muscle mass and repair tissues in the body. The immune system also relies on o sufficient quantity and quality of sleep. Sleep deficiency is therefore linked to difficulty in fighting infection and an increased risk of sickness.

Moreover, research has shown that adequate sleep improves memory and learning, increases attention and creativity, and aids in making decisions. Hence sleep deprivation con noticeably affect performance, including one's ability to think clearly, react quickly, or form memories.

Sleep deprivation also affects mood, leading to irritability and problems with relationships – especially for children and teenagers – and increased anxiety.

Sleep disturbances may be a sign of some mental health challenges, especially depression and anxiety disorders. Indeed, lock of sleep is a common trigger for mental illness. Lost but not least, sleep deprivation increases the risk of developing dementia.

Hence, adequate sleep is important to both preventing the onset of illness as well as preventing a relapse.

So what would constitute adequate good quality sleep? The Prophet's sleep routine would be the ideal model for us to follow:

> "One *should not sleep before the night prayer, nor have discussions after it*"
> —[Hadith, Bulchari}

In other words, go to bed soon after lshaa' prayer (about 9pm).

Also, avoid doing any stimulating activity like having conversations (online or otherwise) during the time before bed. The Prophet (saw) also had a night time routine of darkening his room and making *du'a* (supplications) before he slept. Recent research has shown that this is a good thing to emulate: a regular non-stimulating bedtime routine enhances our sleep quality.

Fact: Sleep-deprived people who were tested using a driving "'Il simulator or performing hand-eye coordination tasks did as badly as, or worse than, people who were intoxicated. Drowsy driving causes thousands of road accidents each year, some of .._ them fatal.

CHAPTER 13

The Sun, the Earth and Fresh Air

8 Here comes the sun...and I say it's alrigh-H."

—*The Beatles*

The sun

A direct health benefit of being in the sun is in the production of Vitamin 03. Among children, lack of Vitamin D due to lack of sun may result in a condition called rickets, where the bone becomes fragile and fractures easily. Too much sun is also bad, especially in lighter skinned people where the risk of developing a skin cancer known as melanoma increases. Australia has one of the highest incidences of melanoma in the world, given the popular practice of sunbathing by the white population.

The ear1h

Research has shown that walking barefoot on grass, sand, soil or rock can reduce pain and fatigue. When our bare feet comes into contact with the earth, free electrons ore token up into the body. These electrons ore nature's biggest anti-oxidants that help neutralize free radicals and hence reduce inflammation. So go ahead, remove your shoes and walk the earth! But do take care not to step on broken gloss or other things that can harm you. Better still, help remove these when you come across them.

> .. and removing harmful things from the path
> is an act of charity."
> —[Hadith, Bulchari]

Fresh air

Fresh air containing oxygen is necessary for all human activity, as it is used to break down sugar to produce energy for our muscles. The more active we are, the more oxygen we need. Unfortunately, air containing pollutants means, as we breathe in oxygen, we may also pollute our lungs. Most Singaporeans become painfully aware of the importance of fresh air when we experience the haze that arises from forest fires in neighbouring countries. Not only people with lung conditions such as asthma suffer, but also healthy individuals. The haze also results in the rise of other conditions such as allergic rhinitis and allergic conjunctivitis. When people remain indoors to avoid the ill-effects of the haze, they also do less exercise than usual, affecting their health in other ways.

Deep bregthjng god relgxqtjon

The deep breathing and relaxation technique is a technique that has been introduced in recent years to help maintain good health. Among its benefits are:

- Relief of stress and tension
- Improved oxygenation in tissues
- Improved immunity
- Removal of toxins
- Increased energy levels

> 0Pians to protect air and water, wilderness and wildlife are in fact plans to protect man."
> —Stewart Udall

CHAPTER 14

Health Screening

"Just because you're not sick doesn't mean you're healthY"

—Anon

Regular health exams and tests {health screening) con help foresee problems before they start, or at least detect problems early, when chances for treatment and cure ore better. By getting the right screenings, and early treatments, you ore taking steps towards living a healthier life.

The best place to go for health screen is your regular health core provider. For most, it is the family doctor or government polyclinic. Some community organisations, such as SATA or NKF, also conduct health screens.

The types of useful health screenings would be the following:

- *Blood pressure:* age 18 upwards, every two years
- *Urine analysis:* age 18 upwards, every three years
- *Diabetes:* age 40 upwards, every three years
- *Cholesterol:* age 40 upwards, every three years
- *Breast cancer (breast self-examination {"BSE"j):* age 18 upwards, monthly
- *Cervical cancer (Pap Smear}:* sexually active females, every three years
- *Colorectal cancer (stool test):* age 50 upwards, annually
- *Oral health:* every six months from the age of six

For those of us with a family history of certain illnesses, it would be advisable to go for screening earlier. For example, if you have a parent or sibling who developed breast cancer at the age of 40, then it is recommended to go for an additional screening mammogram when you turn 35, even if you do not feel a lump through BSE.

CHAPTER 15

Vaccination

"If everything is Gods will, then so is the invention of the vaccine, just like the seatbelt."

—*Els Borst*

Why is vaccination important?

Experts say that it is the most effective method of preventing infectious diseases such as polio, measles and tetanus.

My medical colleague Dr Iskandar ldris, who volunteered at the 2004

Tsunami in Aceh, shared with me that he was shocked to see many cases of tetanus (a horrible illness where victims go into uncontrollable muscle spasms) due to the lock of access to vaccines there. This year in 2019, there have been cases of measles outbreaks in the US (although back in 2000, measles was eliminated in the US) and other countries. This is the sod consequence of on anti-vaccination drive from those who believe that the measles vaccine can cause autism.

Vaccination is the administration of weakened germs (o vaccine) into a healthy individual to stimulate his immune system to develop immunity to the germ (e.g., the measles virus that causes measles). When o sufficiently Iorge percentage of o population has been vaccinated, herd immunity results, *i.e.,* because less people will be infected on exposure to a sick person, the disease will not spread so fast in the community.

Recommended vaccines

In Singapore, some vaccines are compulsory and given during childhood such as those against tuberculosis, diphtheria, pertussis, tetanus, polio, hepatitis B, measles, mumps and rubella. Others are optional but certainly recommended for all children, including varicella (chickenpox), haemophilus influenza b, rotavirus and pneumococcus.

For girls and young women, before they become sexually active, the vaccine against HPV (Human Papilloma Virus) is recommended to help prevent cervical cancer.

For adults, it is also recommended that we get a booster vaccine for Diphtheria, Pertussis and Tetanus.

The annual influenza vaccine is recommended for at-risk groups such as healthcare professionals, travellers and those with lowered immunity such as people with diabetes and the elderly.

For the frail elderly and others with lowered immunity, the pneumococcal vaccine further helps reduce their chance of contracting pneumonia.

For travellers, various vaccines are recommended, depending on where they are heading. These include vaccines against rabies, meningococcus, Japanese B encephalitis, cholera, typhoid, yellow fever and smallpox.

CHAPTER 16

Health Supplements

"I take a vitamin everyday; if s called a steak."
−Robert Duvall

Quite often, people ask me *to* recommend a health supplement for them. Most are willing *to* spend money *to* help prevent or cure ailments, and are more willing to take supplements than medications.

Our ageing population and a heightened interest in health and wellbeing have helped boost sales of health supplements.

But do we really need any of them?

It's important to remember that supplements are designed to supplement our diet, not to replace nutritious foods.

Foods offer not only vitamins and minerals, but also fibre, nutrients (carbohydrates, proteins, and fats), phytochemicals, and a whole host of nutritious substances.

Still, some people may require supplements because the vitamins and/or minerals they need are hard to get in sufficient amounts in the diet. These groups include:

- Pregnant women
- Nursing mothers
- Strict vegetarians, especially vegans
- Fussy eaters (usually children)
- People with food allergies or intolerances
- Elderly

Multivitamins

There is no harm in taking a once-daily multivitamin, as long as you select one based on your age and gender. For example, the ones for women will contain more iron while those for the elderly will hove more calcium. But better than a multivitamin is to fill in the gaps with food that offers so much more.

Calcium

Calcium is one of the minerals most often locking in our diet. Whenever you can, you should choose calcium from foods such as dairy products, fortified foods, dark leafy greens, soybeans, beans, fish and raisins.

Glucoaamine and Chondroitin

These supplements ore often token by people with joint pain. Some find relief from taking the the combination of glucosamine and chondroitin Glucosamine alone usually does not work.

Fish oil

There is a misconception that fish oils can lower cholesterol. While this is a myth, studies do show that omega-3 fatty acids found in fish oil protect your heart. It is therefore recommended that you consume fatty fish twice weekly. However, it has not been proven that taking a supplement can have the same benefit.

I Complex

The vitamin B complex includes thiamine, niacin, riboflavin, pantothenic acid, vitamin B--6, and vitamin B--12. Many of us don't need these supplements. One exception is the elderly, who may need additional B-12 because as one gets older, less of it is absorbed from food.

VitaminC

Vitamin Cis often taken to help prevent catching a cold, though there is little proof this actually works. But it will not do any harm to take up to about 1 gram daily. Rich food sources of vitamin C include oranges, peaches, papayas, pineapples, broccoli, strawberries, tomatoes and melons.

Vitamin D

Vitamin Dis needed to regulate calcium and phosphate in our blood so that we con maintain healthy bones. It is likely that you ore not getting enough vitamin D if you spend most of your time indoors, as skin exposure to the early morning sun gets our cells to produce vitamin D from cholesterol. If you belong to this group, be sure to eat a variety of foods rich in vitamin D such as fortified milk and cereals, or fish like salmon and tuna. Alternatively, take a daily vitamin D supplement.

The dangers of mega doses

Many consumers go way beyond the daily multivitamin, and take a host of dietary supplements. But is more, better?

NO. In fact, exceeding the Recommended Daily Allowances for some vitamins and minerals could be lethal. For example, overdosing on Vitamin D can result in hypercalcaemia (high calcium blood levels) that con produce symptoms of vomiting, polyuria (producing too much urine), polydipsia (drinking huge amounts due to thirst), encephalopathy (brain swelling) and kidney dysfunction.

Generally, it is safer to toke less than the recommended dose as you would be consuming some of it in your food.

Be especially careful with minerals and fat-soluble vitamins A, D, E and K, as they can build up in your system.

CHAPTER 17

Building Natural Immunity

"'MothetS may breastfeed their children two complete yeatS for whoever wishes to complete the nutSing [period] ..".'
—[Ouran 2:233]

Babies enter this world with on inexperienced immune system. Slowly, children develop their immunity by bottling on ongoing series of genms, which is why six to eight bouts of flu, cold or ear infections per year is nonmol for them.

Nevertheless, there are steps you can take to help boost your children's immune system.

Breaatfeed

Breast milk contains immunity-enhancing antibodies and white blood cells. Breastfeeding guards against ear infections, allergies, diarrhoea, pneumonia, meningitis, urinary tract infections, and sudden infant death syndrome (SIDS). It may also enhance your baby's brain power and help protect him against insulin-dependent diabetes and certain forms of cancer later in life. Colostrum, the thin yellow "pre-milk" that flows from the breasts during the few days after birth, is especially rich in disease fighting antibodies. Mothers should aim to breastfeed for two years. If not achievable, aim to breastfeed for at least the first two to three months in order to supplement the immunity your baby received in the womb.

Fact: Breostfeeding benefits mothers too. It con help reduce the following: womb bleeding after birth; pregnancy weight faster; insulin requirement for mothers with Type 1 diabetes;and the risk of getting breast and ovarian cancer, as well as osteoporosis. It helps the mother bond with her baby better and is certainly ... more economical!

Ensure enough sleep

Sleep deprivation can make a child more susceptible to illness by reducing natural killer cells from the immune system that attack microbes and cancer cells. How much sleep do children need? A newborn may need up to 18 hours daily, toddlers require 12 to 13 hours, and preschoolers need about 10 hours. If your child cannot take naps during the day, try to put him to bed earlier.

Serve mora fruits and vegetables

Fruits and vegetables such as carrots, green beans, oranges and papaya contain phytonutrients such as Vitamin C and carotenoids. These phytonutrients help increase the body's production of white blood cells which help fight infection. They also boost the production of interferon, an antibody that coats cell surfaces and help block out viruses. A diet rich in phytonutrients also helps prevent other diseases as such as cancer and heart disease in adulthood. Our children should eat five servings of fruits and veggies a day. {A serving is about two tablespoons for toddlers and 1 cup for older kids.) Children model after their parents, hence we need to "walk the talk".

Exercise

Regular exercise increases the number of natural killer cells. To get your children into a lifelong fitness habit, be a good role model. Exercise with them rather than just urge them to go outside and play. Fun family activities include bike riding, hiking, basketball, swimming and badminton.

Banish secondhand smoke

Children are more susceptible than adults to the harmful effects of secondhand smoke because they breathe at a faster rate; a child's natural detoxification system is also less developed. Secondhand smoke increases a child's risk of SIDS, bronchitis, ear infections, and asthma. It also affects intelligence and neurological development.

Don't pressure the doctor

It is not advisable to pressure the doctor to write a prescription for an antibiotic whenever your child has a cold, flu or sore throat. Antibiotics treat only illnesses caused by bacteria, but most of childhood illnesses are caused by viruses.

In fact, many doctors prescribe antibiotics somewhat reluctantly at the urging of parents. Strains of antibiotic-resistant bacteria have flourished as a result, and a simple ear infection is more difficult to cure if it is caused by resistant bacteria that do not respond to standard treatment.

I too have felt the pressure of prescribing antibiotics by some parents, and while I have tried to persuade them that antibiotics are not necessary, some can act in a very unpleasant way and continue to pressure me, so much so that I accede to their demands.

Happier and healthier

Give our children the love and attention they need. Happier children, like happier adults, are less likely to fall sick when exposed to germs and even if they do, they get milder symptoms. So let's remind ourselves to keep giving our children the love and attention they need!

CHAPTER 18

Cigareffes

"...do not throw yourselves with your own hands into destruction..."'

−{Our an 2:195}

Spending money on cigarettes is literally uthrowing yourself with your own hands into destruction". Cigarette smoke contains over 4,000 chemicals, including 4 known cancer-causing (carcinogenic) compounds and 400 other poisons including tor (used on roods) and formaldehyde (used to preserve dead bodies). Nicotine in cigarettes make them highly addictive.

Increased health risk

Smoking is estimated to increase the risk of:

- Coronary heart disease by 2 to 4 times
- Stroke by 2 to 4 times

- Lung cancer by more than 25 times **Benefits of quiHing (almost lmmedlatel)** <u>On the body</u>
- Blood circulation improves.
- Less breathlessness and coughing.
- Able to concentrate better and less prone to headaches.
- Have a lower chance of developing lung cancer.

<u>On the appearance</u>

- Less chance of losing teeth, and existing teeth will not stain as easily.
- Hair, eyes, skin and nails will all start to look better.
- Have fresher breath.

<u>On the wallet</u>

1 pack of Marlboro costs $14
$14 x 30 = $420 monthly
$14 x 365 = $5,110 annually ... enough to go for a nice annual vacation!

<u>On the family</u>

Studies have shown that children who live with smokers are several times at greater risk of contracting lung cancer compared with children who live with non-smokers.

Passive smoking increases a non-smoker's risk of lung cancer, heart disease and stroke.

How to control cravings
Exercise

Even moderate physical activity, such as brisk walking, reduces nicotine cravings during and immediately after the activity. Also, endorphins released in the brain will alleviate symptoms of stress (stress is a common reason why smokers continue to smoke).

Cultivate a resilient attitude

Relapses are part and parcel of the process of quitting, so if you relapse, start afresh on your resolution to quit.

Reach out to your loved ones when you are struggling.

Change your ather daily habits

Consider how you can replace your regular smoking routines with healthier activities. For example, if you habitually smoke after dinner, go for a walk instead at that time. Spend time with your family and friends in smoke-free areas. Avoid designated smoking areas.

Help is available!

Quit Line (1800 438 2000} is a toll-free telephone service, staffed by trained quit advisors, which provides support and advice to help smokers quit smoking. It also provides family and friends of smokers with information to help them support the smoker trying to quit.

Reference: Health Promotion Board, Singapore

CHAPTER 19

Alcohol and Gambling

"They ask you about wine and gambling.
Say: 'In them is great sin, and some profit,
for men; but the sin is greater than the profit.'"
—[au;an 2:219]

Alcohol

Alcohol is a brain depressant -that is, it reduces the activity of brain cells. The potential harm from excessive alcohol consumption is numerous.

- *Behavioural:* family, employment, or legal problems; injury due to domestic abuse, accidents, or violence;marital discord, divorce and low academic achievement.
- *Psychiatric:* affective disorders (e.g. depression), personality disorders, comorbid substance use disorders, including tobacco addiction.

- *Medical:* hypertension, gastrointestinal symptoms, abnormal liver enzyme levels, anemia (leading to breathlessness and fatigue), thrombocytopenia (low platelet count leading to increased bleeding risk), osteoporosis, menstrual dysfunction, breast cancer, end stage liver disease.

Alcohol addiction is a primary and chronic disease that is progressive (worsens with time) and often fatal (WHO definition). Sjgns gf glcghol gddjctjgn

- Compulsion to drink
- Pre-occupation with obtaining alcohol
- Needing greater amounts to get the same amount of pleasure from the drink
- Withdrawal symptoms
- Continued use even with visible adverse effects
- Rapid relapse after a period of abstinence

Women are more at risk of alcoholic addiction than men. Also the younger you begin drinking, the greater your chances of becoming an alcoholic. Pregnant women cause harm to their unborn foetus with even small intakes of alcohol. Further, every known benefit of drinking a small amount of wine - *e.g.,* benefit to the heart - can be easily gained through the consumption of fruits rich in anti-oxidants. Hence it is best to avoid alcohol completely, as enjoined by our Creator.

Gambling

Gambling is defined as any activity where a person risks an item of value, such as money or jewellery, on the outcome of an event that is determined mostly by chance.

People tend to gamble for different reasons, including the hope of getting rich quick or as an escape from boredom.

Ggmbling myths

- Gambling is an easy way to make money.
- The outcome of a game can be predicted or controlled.
- The likelihood of winning is higher if gamble more.
- Performing certain rituals or owning special objects will improve chances of winning.
- A "near-win" is a sign that a win is just around the corner.

Problem gambling is more than just about on individual engaging in excessive, out-of-control gambling. Gambling addiction is o form of mental illness that is especially dangerous due to difficulty in detection. For every problem gambler, about eight to ten other people (e.g., their spouse, children, parents, other family members, friends, employers) ore harmed by their gambling.

Harms of excessive gambling

Financial problems: Severe debts or the loss of savings or property may arise as a result of gambling losses. The gambler may even resort to borrowing money or stealing to fund gambling activities.

Relationship problems: Lying or deceit on the part of the problem gambler due to the desire to hide gambling activities may strain relationships.

Physical and mental health: The stress of gambling problems sometimes causes health problems, for both the person who gambles and the family. This can include stress, anxiety, depression and even suicide.

> *8 0 you who believe! Intoxicants and gambling, are an abomination of Satan's handiwork: eschew them so you may prosper. Satan's plan is to excite enmity and hatred between yourselves, with intoxicants and gambling, and hinder you from the remembrance of God, and from prayer: will you not then abstain?"*
>
> —{*Oulan 5:90-91*}

CHAPTER 20

Injuries

"The most frustrating thing about injuries is that they take so bloody long to heal.n
—Joson Statham

Injury is damage to the body caused by external force. This may be caused by accidents, falls, weapons, and so on. Major injury can result in prolonged disability or death.

Injuries are the cause of 9% of all deaths, and are the sixth leading cause of death in the world.

Falls are the leading cause of fatal and non-fatal injuries among the elderly. Falls threaten seniors' safety and independence and generate enormous economic ond personal costs.

To prevent injuries, we need to know the causes.

Why do injuries happen?

Driving beyond speed limit con result in o serious motor vehicle accident; rushing through the lifting of heavy objects may result in serious back injury.

<u>Lack of safety features</u>

The major causes include:

- *For the elderly:* poor lighting, slippery tiles;stairs;worn out soles.

For small children: untested hot water showers or baths; unaccompanied ploy at swimming pools; stairs; unattended cooking implements on stoves.

Carelessness

Looking at the hand phone while driving or walking cause many accidents.

<u>Lack of perception of danger</u>

Both young children and the elderly ore susceptible to this, especially on stairs and roads.

<u>Doing too many things at the same time</u>

Multitasking, *e.g.,* combining babysitting and cooking, is dangerous. For example, a child may enter the kitchen while her mother is frying some chicken and hot oil may splatter on the child.

CHAPTER 21

Sex and Modesty

8 Nor come near to adultery: for it is a shameful (deed) and an evil, opening the road (to other evils}."

—{Our an 17:32}

The consequences of problematic sexual behaviour are well known. Sex outside marriage, for example, often leads to unplanned pregnancies and abortions. Sexual promiscuity leads to the transmission of devastating sexually transmitted diseases such as HIV AIDS, syphilis, herpes, genital warts and gonorrhoea. Infidelity leads to marital problems and eventual divorce, with the subsequent rise in single-parent households.

Sexual abuse of the young often causes PTSD (Post Traumatic Stress Disorder) and the start of mental health issues such as depression and substance abuse.

*"Whenever a man is alone with a woman,
the Devil makes a third"*
—*[Hadith, Tirmidzi}*

The Prophet (saw) has taught us that man's weakness can lead to great sin when left in a vulnerable situation such as a man and a woman being left alone together. Therefore, preventing oneself from being placed in such a situation is of utmost importance. For this reason, the Our'an also advises us not to go anywhere close to committing adultery.

The Our'an describes Satan's mission on earth as follows:

*8 For {SatanJ commands you to do what is
evil and shameful, and to say of God that of
which you have no knowledge."*
—*{Our an 2:169}*

Of course, someone whose actions are guided by Satan will have no shame. A clear example of this is exposure to violence and pornography from the media, and the young particularly is especially vulnerable, no thanks to usocial" media.

*.. if you have no shame, do whatever you
like ..."*
—*[Hadith, Malik]*

Garment of righteousness

> *"0 Children of Adam! We have blessed you with clothes to cover your shame, and to be an adornment for you. But the garment of righteousness, that is the best... Let not Satan seduce you, the way he got your parents out of the garden, stripping them of their clothes, to expose their shame ..."*
>
> *−[Ouran 7:26-27}*

Allah explains to us the importance of covering our shame (private parts). Covering up distinguishes us from other creatures of God, and make us less vulnerable to further indecencies such as free sex. Allah also explains that the best clothes for us are the raiment of righteousness" because it protects us from Satan's seduction.

Lower their gaze and guard their modesty

> *"Say to the believing men that they should lower their gaze and guard their modesty: that will make for greater purity for them: and God is well acquainted with all that they do. And say to the believing women that they should lower their gaze and guard their modesty; that they should not display their beauty and ornaments except what (must ordinarily) appear thereof; that they should draw their head coverings over their bosoms (as well) ...*
>
> *−[Oulan 24:30-31}*

The key to preventing problematic sexual behaviour lie in the above verses. Believing men and women are advised to lower their gaze, that is, to avoid looking at anything that may stimulate unlawful sexual desire. It is natural to want to gaze at an attractive man or woman, especially if their clothes reveal aspects of their physical body that are sexually arousing. While it is easy to blame another for their provocative clothes, Allah tells us to take proactive action in protecting ourselves and our mental health by lowering our gaze.

Such self-censorship is even more urgent in today's world, as it is the only way to protect yourself from the pornography that is easily available on the internet. Lowering the gaze is therefore the hallmark of those who wear the ugarment of righteousness".

Apart from visual stimulation, Islam also advocates avoidance of *fitnah* (tests) in other ways:

For example, it is stated:

> ':.. *they should not strike their feet in order to draw attention to their hidden ornaments ..."*
> −{*Oulan 24:31*}

While another hadith declares *"When* one *of you (women)* comes *to the mosque she must not touch perfume."*

While deodorants ore okay, perfumes that oct like pheromones con arouse sexual desire. Even the voice con be o source of attraction, and in the case of the prophet's wives, it was emphasised that they should not speak with on alluring tone:

> ""0 Wives of the Prophet! You are not like any other women: If you do fear (God), be not too sweet of speech, lest one in whose heart is a disease, should be moved with desire: but speak a speech (that is} just."
> −{Oulan 33:32}

In short, the garment of righteousness includes not only modest clothing, but conduct and speech that is modest. These rules are not there to restrict people but to protect them from the negative consequences of unbridled desire on one's physical, emotional and mental health. When we obey them, we do it for our own good.

Prayer restrains from shameful deeds

For the believing men and women, a powerful means of keeping oneself chaste is through performing regular prayer.

> 11Recite what is sent of the Book by inspiration to thee, and establish regular prayer: for prayer restrains from harmful and unjust deeds; and remembrance of God is the greatest (thing in life) without doubt. And God knows the (deeds) that you do."
> −{Our an 29:45}

Marriage

Islam also advocates marriage partly because within a marriage, the sexual needs of individuals can be met the *halal* way. Many young couples delay marrying due to financial reasons. One way this burden can be reduced is to keep the wedding ceremony as simple as possible.

> *"The marriage which receives more blessing*
> *is that which involves less burden."*
> — {*Hadith, Baihaqi*}

CHAPTER 22

IQ, EQ, SQ- Our Three Main Intelligences

(Aqal, Akhlaq, Taqwa)

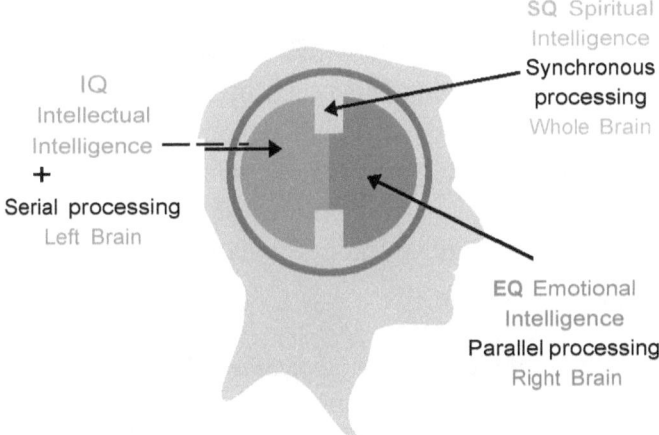

Three dimensions

The diagram above illustrates the three dimensions of intelligence, corresponding to intellectual intelligence

(10}, emotional intelligence (EO), and spiritual intelligence (SO).

10, or intelligence quotient, is the score derived from one of several standardized tests designed to assess an individual's intelligence.

Emotional Intelligence, or emotional quotient (EO), is defined as an individual's ability to identify, evaluate, control, and express emotions.

A 2007 meta-analysis found that emotional intelligence was associated with better mental and physical health.

Spiritual Intelligence (SO) is defined as:

"The intelligence with which we address and solve problems of meaning and value, the intelligence with which we can place our actions and our lives in a wider, richer, meaning-giving context, the intelligence with which we can assess that one course of action or one life-path that is more meaningful than any other." - *Paul Chippendale, Mjnessence*

Internqtiqnql Coopemtiye {December 2001)

SO is developed primarily through reflection.

Whereas 10 is rule-based, EO helps us act appropriately within society's prescribed boundaries, and SO helps us extend and change the boundaries, question our assumptions and formulate new meaning. It is the intelligence of creativity.

People of higher 10 ore more likely to have the knowledge and skills needed to maintain good health. However, those of higher EO are able to communicate better with others and ward off most stressors – the source of much anxiety and ill-health.

The ultimate winners however are those with higher SO because they remain motivated to stay well and healthy stemming from their clear aims and direction in life.

Hence, it is wise for each of us to develop and nurture all three domains of human intelligence. believe the Islamic equivalents of *10, EO* and SO are *Aqal, Akhlaq* and *Taqwa* respectively.

Aqal (Wisdom)

Aqal is the power of thinking and logic. It discovers unknown realities through the known ones. Wisdom makes logical rules using plausible reasoning by induction and deduction. Wisdom then reaches useful conclusions based on these logical rules.

There are several synonyms used for wisdom in practice including but not limited to reason, intellect, insight, clarity, comprehension, foresight, good judgment and shrewdness. The most prevalent antonyms of wisdom are ignorance and stupidity.

*"Surely the worst of beasts in God's sight
are those that are deaf and dumb and do not
reason."*

—{Our' an 8:22}

Of course, it is obvious that the Our'an does not mean the physically deaf and dumb, but those who do not want to listen to the truth, or those who, when they hear, do not wish to admit it with their tongues. IThe ears that are unable to listen to truth and which are only used for listening to absurd and nonsensical things are deaf. The tongue that utter nonsense is dumb. The people who do not reason ore those who do not make use of their wisdom and their faculty of thought. The Our'an likens them to beasts.

Akhlaq (Conduct)

Akhlaq is the ethics, good conduct and moral character of a person.

*"The only reason why I am sent is to perfect
good akhlaq."*

—[Hadith, Malik]

An act of goodness is much dearer to Allah than one's wealth and richness. Goodness comes from good *akhlaq.*

Good *akhlaq* helps improve our relations with those whom we do not get on;makes us want seek forgiveness from those who are angry with us, and helps create a feeling of brotherhood. The sign of a good person is that his *akhlaq* is excellent.

Taqwa (God conscious)

Taqwa means a lot more than just piousness: it is the fear of incurring Allah's displeasure by making sure that we do what Allah has commanded us to do (for example performing solat and giving zakat) and to avoid what Allah has forbidden (Allah knows best what is not good for His Creation). It is the key to our success in this world and the next.

> *"'0 ye who believe! Fear God and be with those who are true (in word and deed).n*
> —{*Our an 9:119*}

CHAPTER 23

Prayer

•o you who have believed, seek help through patience and prayer. Indeed, Allah is with the patient."

−{Our' an 2:153}

One of Allah's undisputed attributes is that He is Ash-Shafee, the One Who Heals. Believing in Him entails belief that prayer is powerful in preventing illnesses as well as in healing.

This does not mean that we skip our diabetes medicine or refuse a heart by-pass.

"Allah has sent down the disease and the cure, and has made for every disease the cure. So treat sickness, but do not use anything haram."

−[Hadith, Abu Dawood]

Tangible benefits of solat

The daily five compulsory prayers in the life of a Muslim is more than just meditation sessions. Prior to the prayer itself, the practice of ablution does not just clean us physically, but also helps clear the mind and readies the heart for communication with God.

The actual acts of *solat* involve gentle stretching and movement of practically every important muscle in the body, including those in our fingers and toes!

Additionally, the prayer exercises our cognitive skills as we recite the Qur'an from memory, attempting at the same time to pay attention to what the verses mean.

Most of all, prayer promises spiritual healing.

God is near- don't despair

Have you ever fallen so deep into despair that you feel that there is none can come to your aid?

> .lilt was We Who created man, and We know what dark suggestions his soul makes to him: for We are nearer to him than (his) jugular vein."
>
> −{Oulan 50:16}

> For those who believe and worship Allah, they know who to turn to. ""You alone do we worship, and Your aid alone do we seek."
>
> −{Oulan 1:5]

There is no necessity to schedule an appointment to meet Allah.

In our daily prayers, we get to talk to Allah regularly and Allah talks to us each time we read the AI-Ouran and understand its meaning.

Allah has promised:

'When My servants ask ... concerning Me, (tell them) I am indeed close:

> */listen to the prayer of every supplicant when he calls on Me. Let them listen to My call, and believe in Me, so that they will walk in the right way."*
>
> *—{Oulan 2:186}*

When you call upon God to help you, and are willing to listen to Him, Allah guarantees that He will respond. He hears you and He will help you.

The concept of obedience

Regular solat is a training in being constantly and willingly obedient to Allah, because that is how we access His assured help. The Our'an elaborates on the things we need to do to show our obedience to

Him, but they are not onerous. The most important include:

- Being good to one's parents

- Avoiding shameful deeds
- Being trustworthy
- Being just

> "... Join not anything as equal with Him; be good to your parents; kill not your children for fear of poverty – we provide sustenance for you and for them; do not go near shameful deeds, openly or in secret; take not life, which God has made sacred, except by way of justice or law: thus does He command you, that you may learn wisdom. Also, do not approach an orphan's property, except to improve it, until he attains the age of full strength; and give measure and weight justly ... Whenever ye speak, speak justly, even if a near relative is concerned ... Thus does He command you, that ye may remember."
>
> *–[Ouran 6: 151-152}*

In other words, the same things that make you a good person are the things you need to do to obey God. He does not make it difficult for us to reach Him.

The concept of Tawakkal

> 8 On no soul does Allah place a burden greater than it can bear"
>
> *–[Ouran 2:286}*

Furthermore, Allah has promised that we will never be given a challenge that we cannot cope with.

Nevertheless, to keep the mind, body and soul healthy, prayer must always be accompanied by effort, after which we put our trust in Allah *(tawakka.*

Tawalclcal is o powerful concept whereby emphasis is placed on putting in effort first, then trusting in God for results.

> *"Trust in God, but tie your camel."*
> −*[Hadith, Tirmidhi}*

Conclusion

Allah tells us to seek help from Him in patience ond prayer. Regular prayer is itself on exercise in patience. And prayer with trust ond conviction is promised results. In short, if you do your prayers regularly, it will help you achieve oil your goals, especially the ones that relate to your well-being. So start establishing regular prayer today - it is on integral port of o truly healthy lifestyle.

CHAPTER 24

Effective Communication

'When you are greeted with a greeting, greet with one better than it or return it in a like manner."

−{Ouran 4:86}

"Spread the greeting of peace among yourselves"- [Hadith, Bukhari} MAssalamu'alaikum!"

−Peace be upon you!

'Wa'alaikumussalam Wa Rahmatullahi Wa Barakaatuh"- And upon you be Peace and the Mercy of God and His Blessings!

The exchange of "Salam" is o universal practice among Muslims that can effectively break barriers and foster relationships if done mindfully. It is not only a greeting of peace but an obligatory prayer for the people you meet, so it is simply not possible to soy it with malice or anger in the heart. When we are mindful of the Salam, we are prompted to push away any negative feelings and re-establish good relationship with the people around us. And the ones we greet ore obliged to return the greeting of peace, and they are encouraged to improve the greeting by invoking the mercy and the blessing of God upon the greeter.

All our communications with others should be modelled upon this - say things to make people feel loved, and respond to the greetings/ good wishes of others with even better words. Good words do not mean meaningless flattery- they should reflect our sincere wishes for others. More importantly, our hearts should be moulded to regularly wish others well.

Communication is o two-way process and to be effective, it should be done in a way that conveys elements of respect, attention and love.

When two people communicate, the intended meaning may not necessarily be the same as the perceived meaning. When this happens, misunderstanding results.

Otherwise, a breakdown in communication can happen, be it between family members, friends or colleagues. Very often, the breakdown leads to conflicts which contribute to ill-health, especially in the mental and emotional domains.

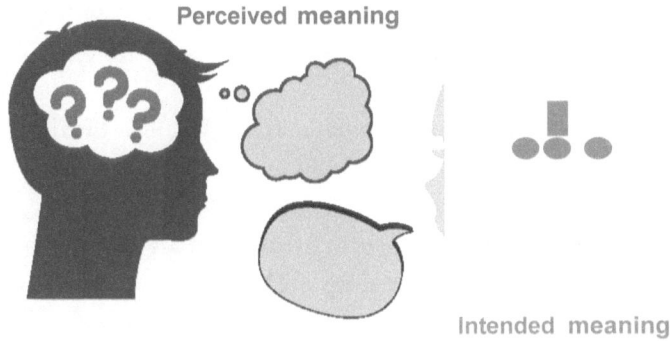

Perceived meaning

Intended meaning

Signala

Research shows that when we communicate feelings and attitudes, only a small percentage of our overall message comes from the words we use. 55% of our message comes from body language, 38% of our message comes from tone of voice, and only 7% of our message is conveyed by the words we use (Mehrabian, 2007).

It is important, therefore, to recognise the "Go" and 11No-Go" signals, that is, behaviour in other people to recognise whether or not they are willing to have a conversation with us.

"Go" signals are when the other person is exhibiting one or more of the following moods:pleasant, happy, excited, cheerful, friendly and calm.

The "No-Go" signals include the following: anger, preoccupation, agitation or tiredness.

The "Mayben (50:50) signals are as follows: sadness, boredom, frustration, depression, shyness or loneliness.

(Reference: *Effective Communication Module,* Healing Friends Training, Club HEAL)

Basic principlee of communication Keep the message short, clear and simple. Do this in a conducive environment.

And if we have said something hurtful, apologise quickly, respectfully and sincerely.

Transference

Transference is the set of expectations, beliefs and emotional responses that a person brings to a relationship. It is based on repeated experiences a person has had with other people throughout life. Hence it is very important to "not take it personally" if a stranger dislikes you for no apparent reason. It could be because you remind him of someone for whom he has a great dislike.

Empathy

Empathy is a very important quality that allows a person to successfully engage with and win the confidence and trust of another person. It is the intimate comprehension of another person's thoughts and feelings "Putting ourselves in that person's shoesn. It helps to avoid or diffuse conflict.

In order to empathise, we need to be able to actively listen to what another person is saying, an excellent technique can help us to not only understand what that person is going through but also making him feel that the we ore genuinely interested and sincere in helping.

Important tips for parents and teachers:

- *Don't criticise:* Try to understand and empothise instead
- *Don't pressure:* Simply encourage and support
- *Don't judge:* Let Allah be the Judge
- *Don't* males *comparisons:* Each person is special and has his/her own strengths

Manage own expectations- expectations are added sources of stress and anxiety.

Lastly, let us ponder upon the following statement by someone very dear to me, giving a fresh new perspective to the term Hfrom heart to heart":

> *"People think it is only through words that pass your lips and your body language that information and love can be communicated. They do not realise that the most powerful way of disseminating information to every single human is through the heart."*
>
> *−/man Harharah*

CHAPTER 25

Work and Studies

*"The highest reward for man's toil is not what
he gets for it, but what he becomes by it."*
—John Ruskin

Work and studies *can* help prevent a person from
becoming unwell and unhealthy. This is provided that
the undertaking matches the person's interest and ability
and is meaningful.

Otherwise, work or studies can trigger illness due to the
stress and anxiety it brings to the person.

For example, when parents force their child to take up
a course of study that their child is not interested in or
have no aptitude for, the child is likely to fall sick often
due to emotional and mental strain. He is also more
likely to drop out of the course of study.

When on employer foils to match his employees to the right kind of work, either their well-being will be affected, or they will leave the company to preserve their health.

The importance of creating a conducive work environment can never be understated. This includes fair working hours, o just system of rewards and benefits, and good communication between employer and employees, as well as fellow employees. Employers must be open to flexible work schedules and hove the interests of their employees at heart to gain the respect and loyalty of their employees.

A healthy work environment is good not just for the health of the employees but also for the health of the whole organisation, because healthier and happier staff are also more productive.

Yet not everyone is cut out for employment; for those who prefer to be their own bosses- just do it even if it means sacrificing some material security.

Work then become a pleasure rather than a chore. And if that endeavour is accompanied by the sincere wish to serve Allah, it will certainly yield the best rewords.

> *"Deeds are evaluated by intentions, and a person will get the reward according to his intention ..."*
>
> *—[Hadith, Bukhari}*

CHAPTER 26

Sports and The Arts

"That awe, wonder and beauty promote healthier levels of cytokines suggests the things we do to experience these emotions – a walk in nature, losing oneself in music, beholding art - has a direct influence upon health and life expectancy."

—Dacher Keltner

Both the pursuit of sports and the arts can help prevent illnesses from developing and promote good health. They can be individual pursuits whereby one hones one's hobby and interest or group activities that promote human interaction.

Sports (see also chapter 11 on exercise)

Aisha (ra) stated that:"'*I raced with the Prophet and I beat him. Later, when I had*

> *put on some weight, we raced again and
> he won. Then he said, "This cancels that
> (referring to the previous race.)"*
>   *—[Hadith, Bulchari]*

There is a lot of scientific evidence on the positive eHects of sport and physical activity as part *of* a healthy lifestyle. The positive, direct eHects of engaging in regular physical activity are particularly so in the prevention of several chronic diseases, including cardiovascular disease, diabetes, hypertension, obesity, depression and osteoporosis.

Nevertheless, not all sports are suitable for everyone - we need to be discerning.

For example, for people with early joint pain, some sports, including tennis, badminton and basketball, can worsen the condition. Even for those without arthritis, such sports should be combined with non weight-bearing activities such as swimming and cycling. Triathlons therefore make more sense than marathons.

The Prophet (saw) himself encouraged various sports, including archery, racing, horse riding and swimming. The last is especially useful as an exercise as it strengthens muscles and help build endurance without adversely affecting our joints. Muslim women have no reason to hold back, as covering our *aurah* while swimming is now quite easily achieved, and the health benefits ore immeasurable.

Tile Arts

> HAllah, the Most High, is beautiful and
> likes beauty."
>
> —[Hadith, Muslim]

The Arts refer to the creation of works of beauty or other special significance.

Artistic expression is the conscious use of the imagination in the production of objects intended to be contemplated or appreciated as beautiful, as in the arrangement of forms, sounds or words.

Apart from painting, artistic activities include culinary art, dance, music, handicrafts, drama, photography, pottery and writing. An appreciation of nature and art boosts the immune system by lowering levels of chemicals that cause inflammations that can trigger diabetes, heart attacks and other illnesses.

Some Muslims sometimes look down on the Arts as useless and even rule it as *haram* (forbidden in Islam).

This needs to change.

While some supposedly artistic expression may be undoubtedly *haram,* placing o blanket bon on certain forms of art such as drama, music and dance is to turn our back on much of the blessings of God that comes in the form of aesthetic appreciation. It is much better to turn to the basic principles of what is *haram* and *halo/to* judge what our boundaries should be when exploring various arts. During the time of the Prophet (sow), he encouraged percussions at weddings, and sword dancing for entertainment, because they were port of contemporary cultural expressions then. Surely, our appreciation of the Arts need not be limited to what the Prophet (sow) allowed during that period alone. In my opinion, ballet and dramas need not be considered un-lslomic if dancers and actors ore allowed to wear clothing that covers the ouroh.

Hence, let the artists/artistes among us strive to develop their passions in o way that conform to Islamic principles. And for the rest of us, let us strive to be less judgmental!

CHAPTER 27

Volunteering

'Whoever looks after the affairs of his brother, Allah will look after his affairs."
−[Hadith, Bulchari}

"Do not underestimate any good deed, even if it is only meeting your brother with a cheerful face."
−[Hadith, Muslim]

The inherent joy in giving makes it a clear candidate as a positive lifestyle choice. In fact, even a sincere smile is a type of giving. Giving of your time or effort to help or bring cheer to others is called volunteering.

I still remember, while in school, how happy I was when my teacher rewarded me with a smile just because I helped her carry student notebooks that she needed to mark.

The joy we receive from volunteering, nevertheless, depends greatly on our sincerity.

Islam encourages us to give for the sake of Allah, expecting a reward from Him alone. For example, Rasululloh (saw) described sincere alms giving as when a person gives with his right hand without his left hand knowing.

When we give with the hope of attaining a worldly reward, we may not always get what we wish for. Even gratitude from the one who receives your help may not always be forthcoming. When this happens, the giver may feel bitter.

On the other hand, if we give with the hope of Allah's reword, Allah promises us He is *Shalcuurun* (Appreciative). We are assured of a generous return from Him, in this world and the Hereafter.

Allah points the picture of those who give sincerely and those who do not os follows:

> -"O *you who have believed, do not invalidate your charity with reminders or injury as does one who spends his wealth [only] to be seen by the people and does not believe in Allah and the Last Day. His example is that of a {large] smooth stone upon which is dust, and which is hit by a downpour that leaves it bare. They {the stones) are unable {to keep]*

anything of what they have earned. And
Allah does not guide the rejectors."

−*{Oulan 2:264}*

-*"And the example of those who spend their*
wealth seeking means to the approval of
Allah and assuring [reward for] themselves is
like a garden on high ground which is hit by
a downpour − so it yields its fruits in double.
And {even] if it is not hit by a downpour,
then a drizzle [is sufficient]. And Allah sees
everything you do."

−*{Quian 2:265]*

Whileas humans we naturally expect acknowledgement from those around us, we should guard that our wish for praise or reward from others does not exceed the intention for acceptance from Allah so that the motivation to give never dies.

The health benefit. of volunteering

We learn to be grgtefyl

When we help others overcome their stressful times, we will be exposed to o world different from ours. The people we help may be faced with challenges that we ourselves have not experienced, be they challenges in communication, possessions, health or other stuff. That way, we are more mindful of the blessings God has given us.

"Look at the people beneath you (in wealth and worldly aHairs) and do not gaze upon the ones above you (in this matter). This way, you will not underestimate the bounty of Allah bestowed upon you."- [Hodith, Bukhari]

We learn to be bymble

Sometimes other people face challenges that are more destructive than what we face. However, they may show more patience and resilience than us. When we reflect upon their reaction and compare that to our own responses towards challenges that are not as difficult as theirs, we learn to be humble - and we too ore inspired to be just as tough when we face our own challenges.

Self-esteem boosted

When others appreciate our help, or have experienced relief or benefited through our assistance, we will naturally be proud of ourselves. Our ability to make a difference in the lives of our fellow humans will raise our self-esteem and make us feel appreciated. That is why volunteering is a win-win situation.

We forget oyr own wprrjes

Too much time spent on analysing our own problems may worsen our level of anxiety. In contrast, helping others out of their difficulties will help us forget our own worries, albeit temporarily. It allows us to pause and later come back to our own problems with a fresh perspective, which is always useful.

Conclusion

When we look at our problems, we often wonder, "Why must I be tested like this?" We see ourselves as needing help, instead of seeing ourselves in the position to serve others. However, you will be pleasantly surprised by the positive effects that emerge from helping others.

Just remember not to focus on what we will gain when deciding to help others. We do not need any excuse to help, apart from the sincere intention to please God. The truth is that when we do this, we benefit as much if not more than those whom we help. And we ore investing in the hereafter at the same time.

So let us do what we con to support those in need. HEAL ...and be healed!

CHAPTER 28

The Best Things in
Life are Free

*"My father would lift me high. And dance
with my mother and me and then. Spin me
around till/ fell asleep. Then up the stairs
he would carry me and I knew for sure I
was loved."*

—*Luther Vandross*

Many assume that without money life would be
miserable as they will have to forego the good things
in life. The truth is, however, the more things you want
to purchase, the more money you need.

I have good news.

The best things in life are free! Or almost ...

We hear people say, uMoney is not everything but everything needs money". Also,"There is no such thing as a free lunch."

Well, I beg to differ.

Here is a list of the top seven best things in life that are free! Or almost ...

- The air we breathe costs nothing.
- Water that rehydrates costs next to nothing.
- Sleep recharges and refreshes.
- A sincere smile chases the blues away.
- A bear hug takes away tiredness.
- Exercise is invigorating.
- Prayers provide solace.

I hope to convince you that these are seven things that most can acquire, regardless of the amount we earn, and that they are indeed among the best things in life!

Fresh air

Notice how upset we get whenever we experience the haze in Singapore? Rush to buy masks to protect their airways. We think twice before leaving the house. For those who have lung ailments such as asthma or chronic obstructive lung disease, anxiety set in, medical bills soar, medical leave need to be taken. Only one good thing emerges for the smokers, they hove o good reason to quit smoking!

How wonderful it feels when the haze is brought under control and we con breathe fresh air again!

Also, I recall what my late mum said when we went for a holiday to Australia; she remarked how clear and dry our mucus was compared to the dark, sticky ones we had when in Singapore! She made me laugh but it also mode me think, yes, snot from the nose was o rather accurate indicator of air pollution.

Hence, let us all ploy our port to protect the wonderful fresh air we have by reducing the use of things that can pollute it.

Bregtbjng

The way we breathe is important as it can enhance our enjoyment of the air we inhale, especially for those who suffer from anxiety or panic attacks. Anxiety may, among other things, cause one to breathe too fast and too much, such that a chemical imbalance occurs in our bloodstream. Hyperventilation causes excessive carbon dioxide to be exhaled, causing the person to experience headache, weakness, chest pain and numbness and cramps in their hands and feet.

How do we manage a panic attack? Learn how to breathe as follows:

- Sit or lie down
- Inhale slowly and deeply through the nose
- Exhale slowly through the mouth

- Repeat several times.

Soon, the hyperventilation will cease and the feeling of panic will dissipate.

Clean water

Water is the source of life for all living things on this earth.

> *"And have you seen the water that you drink? Is it you who brought it down from the clouds, or is it We who bring it down? If We willed, We could make it bitter, so why are you not grateful?"*
>
> *−{Qur' an 56:68-70}*

Imagine someone falling from a plane to the ocean, and fate has it that he is floating on the sea with a lifejacket - water, water, everywhere but not a drop to drink!

Try to visualise just how good water tastes each time we break our fast during Ramadhan or we quench our thirst during a hot day.

Nutrition experts almost unanimously agree that the best drink for our health is water. If we practice drinking water, this will not only improve our health but also help us save on spending.

I am grateful that these days, most wedding functions provide *'sky* juice'.

Some people claim they are so busy they have no time to hydrate themselves, or they fear drinking water because they cannot spare the time to relieve themselves. No! They put themselves at risk of getting conditions such as kidney stones, gout, urinary tract infections as well *as constipation.*

Showers god gblytjgn

ulf you ore angry, perform ablution with water"- [Hodith, Nowowi]

When we ore angry or sleepy or tired after working all day long, isn't it simply wonderful to immerse ourselves in clean water? Both tiredness and other negative feelings will subside.

Warning: Fresh air and fresh water will no longer be free if we continue abusing our planet earth. The amount of plastics that we use, the wastage of water, the burning of trees and forests: Every little thing that we do to save or destroy our planet has on impact. So please reuse and recycle, and ovoid disposable cutlery, *etc.*

Mother Earth needs each of us to do the right thing by her.

Sleep

I still remember, while performing the hoj in the holy land, we walked at night from Muzdolifoh towards Mino. During our journey I sow many people fast asleep on the streets, with only a mot and a thin blanket. I compare this with others who hove the luxury of a king-sized bed and a comfortable mattress, but still hove trouble sleeping.

Could it be due to mental anguish that their thoughts and emotions ore not able to settle even temporarily so they con enjoy a restful sleep? Or due to overeating, that their stomachs do not allow their minds to rest? Or could it be that the owner of the huge bed is simply not tired enough to need rest? Or did he drink too much coffee during the day time to remain alert, and as a result cannot sleep at night? hospital workers or security officers on night shift duty - many of them have their health affected. They sacrifice their sleep to perform their duties. Hence, if you have the choice, it is far better to avoid doing shift work.

> *"And We make your sleep as a thing for rest,*
> *and We make the night as clothing ..."*
> *−[Quian 78:9- 10]*

Fortunate is he who is able to sleep well after a hard day's work. Night is compared to clothing because he who sleeps undisturbed at night and wakes up to a new day is like one who has received new clothes to replace his dirty old ones, giving him a freshness to commence his duties.

A sincere smile

> *"A smile for your brother is charity"*
> *−[Hadith, Tirmidzi]*

It has also been narrated in another hadith that the Prophet (saw) was one who smiled often.

Why are we encouraged to smile?

Indeed, a smile often begets another smile in return and this will make both parties happy because a smile reflects the happiness within the giver, and, simultaneously, the feeling is then shared.

Smjle tbemP¥

Studies has also shown that it is physically easier for someone to smile than to frown. Other studies have also shown that people who are encouraged to smile are happier than those who are not. people with depression are encouraged to smile to remove negative feelings.

I still remember one morning when I held open the lift door to allow a woman to enter the lift and she rewarded me with a grateful smile - and that gave me a wonderful start to the day. Most people would only say thank you, and there are others who will not even say anything.

Wouldn't it be wonderful if people smile more?

A bear hug

According to studies, there are five reasons why hugging is encouraged:

- It makes a person feel happy and loved
- It reduces a person's blood pressure
- It relieves feelings of anxiety, even if the thing that is hugged is a teddy bear
- It lowers our heart rata
- It lowers our stress levels

Let us give our elderly loving hugs, as they need them even more because of their growing insecurities as they age. Similarly shower infants with hugs; they will grow up to be more confident adults.

Exercise

The benefits of exercise and how to exercise has been discussed in an earlier chapter. The good news is that we do not need to spend much in order to obtain these benefits.

Cheap ActiveSg gym memberships and pool entry fees are affordable for most people. And permanent residents and Singapore citizens are even given grants to buy these without spending your own money. The only cash outlay would be for a proper pair of shoes and comfortable clothes, which would be useful at all times, not just during exercise.

Prayers

During the five daily prayers, we have the opportunity to talk to Allah and Allah speaks to us each time we read the Our'an and reflect upon its meaning. More about this is found in the chapter on Prayer.

> *"Allah, the Most High, says,'I am present when My servant thinks of Me, and I am with him when he remembers Me. If he remembers Me inwardly I shall remember him inwardly. And if he remembers Me among people, I shall remember him among people, who are better than them."'*
>
> *−{Hadith, Bulchari}*

Conclusion

I hope to have convinced you that these are seven things that anyone can have, no matter how little they earn, and that truly these are the best things in life!

Oh yes, one last thing: a lunch treat by a beloved friend is always extra delicious!

CHAPTER 29

Laughter

"A good Iough heals a lot of hurts."
—Madeleine L'Engle

I used to read the Reader's Digest in my younger days and my favourite section was "Laughter is the best medicine". When reading newspapers, after scanning the headlines, I would go to the cartoon pages to have a good laugh. I have grown more serious over the years, yet my favourite reading material is still Garfield.

Laughter is a basic human need.

Benefits of laughter

Humour and laughter help to not only lighten our mood but also induce positive physical changes in our body.

Short-term benefits

Laughter enhances our intake of air; stimulates our heart, lungs and muscles; and promotes the release of endorphins (natural painkillers) from our brain.

It stimulates circulation and aids muscle relaxation, both of which soothe tension.

A hearty Iough fires up and cools down our stress response, making us feel relaxed.

Long-term benefits

Laughter generates positive thoughts and feelings that bring about the release of neurotransmitters (brain chemicals) that counteract stress and potentially more serious illnesses such as cancer by improving our immune system as a whole.

It helps ease pain by causing the body to release its own natural painkillers (endorphins).

It assists in coping with difficult situations and connecting better with others.

The Prophet's example

A man came to the Prophet and wanted to give him a ride on his camel. The Prophet replied: '*We* should give you a ride on a baby camel then." The man asked, *uo* Messenger of Allah, how can I ride on o baby camel?" The Prophet replied:uAre not all camels the babies of a mother camel?"

These and other examples show that the Prophet Muhammad (saw) was warm-hearted and friendly and he made jokes, especially with word ploy. His gentleness is referred to in the Holy Ouron:

> *"It was by a mercy from God that, you (0 Messenger) were lenient with them. Had you been harsh and hard-hearted, they would surely have scattered away from about you."*
> *—[Ouran 5:159]*

However, when he did make jokes and pleasantries, he always behaved moderately as he did in every aspect of his life. For example, as related by Abu Hurairah, when some of his companions asked, *uo*

Messenger of Allah, you joke with us?" He replied: "Yes, I do. But I only tell the truth." Hence, the most important thing about a joke is that they should not be based on lies.

Also, the Our'an warns us against mocking each other. So, remember to not Iough ot the expense of others; laugh with them.

> o you *who have believed, let not a people ridicule [another1people; perhaps they may be better than them; nor let women ridicule [other 1 women; perhaps they may be better*

> *than them. And do not insult one another*
> *and do not call each other by [oHensive1*
> *nicknames..".*
>
> —{*Oulan 49:111*

Lastly, some forms of humour are not appropriate, and we need to use our judgement to discern a good joke from a bad one. For God does not like those who indulge in lewd acts, and that includes crude humour.

CHAPTER 30

Resilience

•How amazing is the affairs of a believerl. Everything turns out well for him; and that applies only to a believer. If happiness befalls him, he gives thanks to Allah and it turns out well for him, and if an ordeal befalls him, he shows endurance and it turns out well for him."

– [Hadith, Muslim]

To stay healthy, one needs to build resilience. We will then be able to rise above the challenges of modern-day living such os computer screens, plastics, adulterated food and pollution. And even if we do become unwell, we are able to bounce back to wellness in a short period of time ot o lesser cost.

Building Resilience

A resilient mind is by way of world-view and attitude. My formula for resilience is found in the acronym HEAL.

We need to believe that every problem has a solution. This means we do not give up hoping we con recover when we foil ill. Hence, we never stop efforts to recover from any illness.

Emppwerment

Knowledge is power when put into action. Knowledge prepares us to face every challenge. Hence it is important to learn about our illness. After learning, we apply that knowledge in a disciplined manner, by avoiding what we should avoid and doing what we can to mitigate the effects of our illness.

Acceptance

Accept challenges with grace and dignity. Know that it is God that has permitted a challenge to beset you and that He is Most Merciful Most Loving. If He gove it to you, it follows thot, in some woy, it will benefit you, even if you cannot see how. This enables us to face every challenge.

It is easier when everyone is accepting -the person with the illness, his family, the caregiver and the general public, as this will remove barriers and make recovery easier.

A caring community that wants to help a person face challenges starts with the family unit. We should olso extend our love to our friends ond neighbours.

Resilient individuals moke resilient families, which in turn moke resilient

communities.

This is on ideol worth striving for.

> •o *you who believe! Persevere in patience and* constancy;*vie in such perseverance; strengthen each other; and fear Allah; so that you may be successful."*
>
> −*[Ouran 3:200]*

GLOSSARY

ActiveSG- A Sport Singapore portoI with sports news, events calendar os well os facilities ond coaches directory for everyone to watch ond ploy sports

Alhomdulilloh -All Praise be to Allah

Amonoh- Trust

Auroh - Ports of body that needs to be covered by clothing

Du'o- Supplication

Hodith- Traditions of the Prophet Muhammad lnsyo Allah- God willing

lshoo'- Night prayer

MRT- Moss rapid transit (train system in Singapore)

Mino- Place near Mekoh that pilgrims stay during port of hoj Muzdolifoh- Place near Mekoh that pilgrims go through during hoj NKF- Notional Kidney Foundation

Niyyot - Intention

Rosululloh- Messenger of Allah (i.e. Prophet Muhammad) SATA- Singapore anti-tuberculosis association sow - Sollolloohu 'oloihi wossolom - peace be upon him (referring to Prophet Muhammad)

Ustozoh- Female religious teacher

WHO- World Health Organization

ABOUT THE AUTHOR

Dr Radich Salim is the founder and President of Club HEAL,an Institution of a Public Character that was formed in 2012 to promote the healing and recovery of people with mental health challenges. She graduated with MBBS (Hons) from the University of Sydney in 1995,and works as a family physician.

ABOUT THE EDITOR

Noorunnisa d/o PK Ibrahim Kutty is the Hon Secretary of Club HEAL and holds a LL.B (Hons) from the International Islamic University, Malaysia. She has extensive experience editing books,newsletters and articles.